Roberto Carlos Negreiros de Arruda
Éric T. K. C. Mesquita
Karlos Yuri F. Pedrosa

Haematophagous Bats and Rabies in Herbivores

Roberto Carlos Negreiros de Arruda
Éric T. K. C. Mesquita
Karlos Yuri F. Pedrosa

Haematophagous Bats and Rabies in Herbivores

Desmodus rotundus and the Desmondine rage

ScienciaScripts

Imprint

Cover image: www.ingimage.com

This book is a translation from the original published under ISBN 978-3-330-99657-1.

Publisher:
Sciencia Scripts
is a trademark of
Dodo Books Indian Ocean Ltd. and OmniScriptum S.R.L publishing group

120 High Road, East Finchley, London, N2 9ED, United Kingdom
Str. Armeneasca 28/1, office 1, Chisinau MD-2012, Republic of Moldova, Europe
Managing Directors: Ieva Konstantinova, Victoria Ursu
info@omniscriptum.com

Printed at: see last page
ISBN: 978-620-8-59726-9

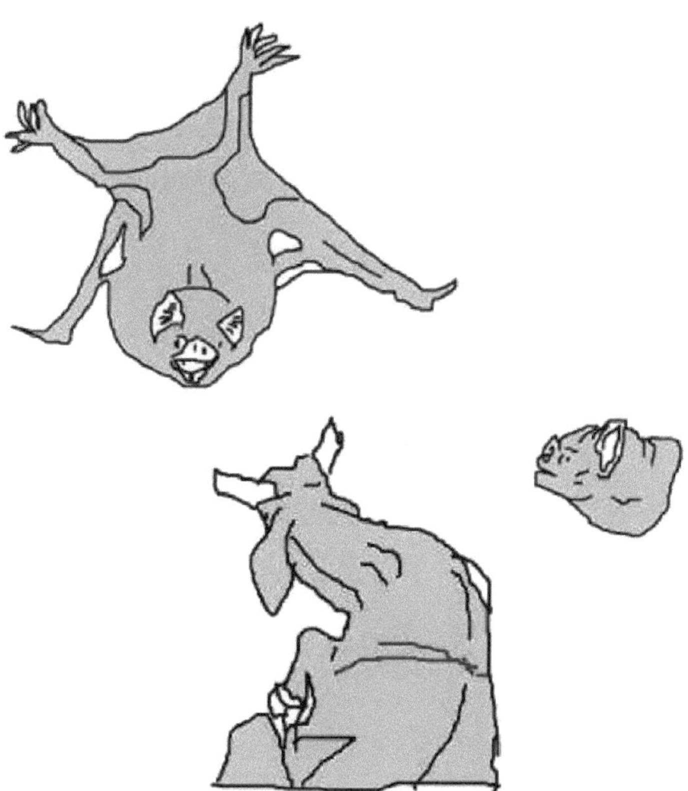

CONTENTS

CHAPTER 1

HAEMATOPHAGOUS BATS AND DESMONDINE RABIES

Roberto Carlos Negreiros de Arruda

The purpose of these explanations is to review the literature on the common vampire, Desmodus rotundus, detailing its biology, demonstrating the risk of disease transmission, highlighting economic losses and providing clarification on the control of this species, as well as relating it to rabies in herbivores.

Rabies is a deadly encephalitis that affects mammals and is best transmitted by animals with more complex dentition (upper and lower teeth), due to contact with saliva. Desmondine rabies transmitted by Desmodus rotundus is a threat to humans, unvaccinated domestic animals and is used to control wild animals due to its mortality rate. However, Desmodus must be infected in order to transmit the disease to those animals that are plundered for food or blood and not to the entire herd, as well as being infected by aggression from other infected bats and not by the blood of an already sick animal. Recently, the potential for spreading the virus to mesocarnivores through the consumption of sick or dying bats has been demonstrated.

In Brazil, the disease is controlled by its main rural transmitter, D. rotundus, either by applying vampiricide to domestic herbivores or paste on the back of bats by teams specialised in capturing, vaccinating animals in rings due to the circular movement of haematophagous bats, and health education is recommended for communities involved in outbreaks of the disease.

Remembering that rabies has other players in the process of spreading over land, including strains or variants that can be carried to other species (spill over), working in partnership between health promotion organisations could be an option for states in controlling the disease.

1. Topics on the bionomics of Desmodus rotundus

- In the world, only three bat species have a haematophagous feeding habit (Desmodus rotundus, Diphylla ecaudata and Diaemus youngi), which are found in Brazil [1];
- In Brazil, there is a report of haematophagous bats being plundered in 1543, when people and animals stayed in Portos dos Reis, in the Pantanal of Mato Grosso 16
- D. *rotundus* females take between 1 and 2 years to reproduce [2] and the gestation period is seven months [3].
- An alpha male has a cluster of females and they are always being challenged by satellite colony males [3], so it is common to find segregation of males and females within the same shelter [4];
- With regard to shelters, caves are not common in regions of dense forests and mangroves[5];
- Tree hollows harbour between 8 and 12 adult bats and a few chicks [2]. In the mangrove swamp, the openings stand out in the siribeira (*Avicennia germinans*) [5];
- Vampire bats housed in wells can be in a small colony, or close to 3 individuals [6].
- The variation in the timing of the appearance of *Desmodus* in more preserved areas may be due to the movement of domestic animals or the deaths of their natural food sources [5]. Similar observations of displacement were made by Costa & Esbérard [7], who in 2011 suggested that *D. rotundus* disperse from the mainland to the islands due to the introduction of domestic animals;
- According to research, D. *rotundus* can live for 12, 6, 18 [32] or 29 years [8];
- To recognise the shelters *of Desmodus* bats, you should look for dark, slimy faeces with an ammoniacal smell [3]. In the case of *Diphylla*, which often shelters in caves, the faeces look like clots and the birds are preferably sucking on the cloaca [9];
- In large shelters (caves) there can be up to 2,000 vampire bats, and it is impossible to capture all the individuals, so if you consider that one bat treated with vampiricides can eliminate 20 others [10], depending on the epidemiology of the disease, you can choose to treat as many as possible to eliminate a greater number of individuals;
- On average, one female joins the main group each year and the males are expelled when

they are around 18 months old [(2)]. These juvenile males look for a new shelter around 3 kilometres from where they were born [11];

- D. *rotundus* uses multiple shelters, generally located in a relatively small area with a radius of 2 to 3 kilometres. These vampires preferentially move along valleys, with males moving more than females [51].
- After two nights without feeding, the bats are starving and close to death. In this situation, the females request regurgitation from their mates, a colony-strengthening procedure known as altruism [2, 15], which is carried out by 70% of mothers or aunts for their young and only 30% of adult females who have failed to feed. In daily foraging, 30% of younger individuals fail to collect blood, and only 7% of adult individuals do so[2];
- Although it is generally assumed that rabies transmission occurs through the bite, laboratory studies have demonstrated the potential for transmission through the ingestion of bat carcasses by mesocarnivores [52];
- In Argentina, as in other areas where bats live, shelters are visited by carnivorous predators to feed on dead or fallen bats. The renewal rate of shelters has been 4 years, with no record of rabies [12]
- Without treatment with the paste, the recolonisation time of daytime shelters by D. *rotundus* was 12.5 months on average, with a variation between three and 25 months [54]
- Naturally, the mortality rate of adult *Desmodus* is around 24 per cent per year[2];

2. Economic losses caused by Desmodus rotundus predation

- The consumption of a small vampire bat is around 20 mL a day and in a year it can reach an impressive 7.5 litres. The elimination of 2,000 Desmodus could represent a balance of 14,990 litres of blood a year, as predicted by Trindad [10];
- Bats can transmit rabies and other pathogens such as trypanosomiasis and cause low milk production in cows. Weight loss per animal reaches 39.7 kg/year and milk loss 1.9 litres per day [12].
- Depredation also causes anaemia, weight loss and death, while the entrance door is prone to myiasis. Desmodus also have the potential to cause diseases in animals and humans such as leptospirosis, brucellosis, equine encephalomyelitis, yellow fever, leishmaniasis, viruses and fungal diseases in their refuge [13, 14];

- In Brazil in 1543, vampire bites caused injuries to humans and caused the deaths of pigs' young due to teat lesions [16]. It is now known that the number of recent attacks on domestic animals is close to the number of bats captured and treated in corrals [5, (11,15)].

3. ***Rabies or rabies virus neutralising antibodies in bats***

- Of the 167 species of chiroptera in Brazil, 41 or 24 per cent were positive for rabies [17]. In São Paulo, 1.9% of all bats were naturally infected [18], showing a low viral load among bats;
- Ruminants do not play an important role in the transmission of the rabies virus, *Desmodus* bats do [6]. In Maranhão, the presence of *D. rotundus* has been shown to increase the likelihood of rabies in domestic herbivores by up to 1.5 times compared to other encephalitis [19];
- Fights between males can be a source of contagion for the rabies virus and the losers can fly up to 100 kilometres away [10];
- Rabies in Argentina produced a high mortality rate in vampires, which exceeded 50% of the population and spread rapidly, after 3 more years without episodes, which extended to 100 kilometres a year. From 1992 to 2001, the mortality of the exposed cattle herd was 0.08% [12] and due to the mortality of transmitters, it is cyclical [19];
- The cohabitation of D. *rotundus* with other bat species favours rabies endemism [20]. *Artibeus* (frugivorous) and *Myotis* (insectivorous) have been observed with the same *variant 3 as Desmodus rotundus* [21];
- Studies in Argentina have reported different patterns of neutralising antibodies and rabies isolation found in vampires in zones classified as epizootic areas (high number of outbreaks), uninfected areas and enzootic areas (number of outbreaks cyclical or in recess). In the area where rabies was in recess, no virus was found in saliva or tissues, but an antibody rate of 24% was found in *Desmodus*. In an epizootic area, 24 per cent of vampire bats were also isolated from rabies virus, but no antibodies were found in their sera. And finally, in the infected area, neither virus nor antibody was detected [33]. Indicating that some of the bats had already died of rabies when the outbreak in herbivores became evident;
- Other studies into the epizootiology of rabies in haematophagous bats were carried out in northern Argentina three years later. In which vampire populations were studied before,

during and after varying intervals of bovine rabies outbreaks. A total of 1,024 *D. rotundus* were examined for antibodies and viruses, while 83 of these were examined only for virus isolation. Neutralising antibodies rarely appear in serum samples obtained before outbreaks of bovine rabies. Of the vampires captured during outbreaks, a low proportion of samples tested positive for antibodies. However, varying proportions of positive samples (including some high rates) were obtained from vampires taken at varying intervals after outbreaks. In this study eleven virus isolations were made, in all cases coming from vampires captured during or shortly before bovine rabies outbreaks [34]. This suggests that a number of bats did not die during the outbreak and that there is a circulating virus and the possibility of a new cycle;

- A capture-recapture study was carried out in 20 colonies of vampire bats, covering four regions of Peru, showing seroprevalence of 3 to 28 per cent, higher in juvenile and sub-adult bats, as a result of adult elimination campaigns 55; Captures and treatments with vampiricides are aimed at the transmission of rabies to herbivores and not to the transmitters, and let's not forget that a proportion of individuals also die of rabies;
- It has been suggested that the rabies virus acts on vampire bat populations in the same way that many other viruses act on other hosts. That is, the virus infects many individuals, some of whom die and others survive, proving their exposure to the virus through antibodies. Over time, the virus disappears from the population of dead vampires, immunity decreases with the density of susceptibles to a value below the contagion threshold and does not return until the incorporation of a number of new susceptibles (either by birth or through the arrival of new bats). The results of these studies indicate that rabies epizootics in haematophagous bats are progressive, always moving in a certain direction. They also tend to have a periodicity of four or more years between outbreaks [35].
- In 1994, it was found that only male individuals of the D. *rotundus* species in the Botucatu/SP region tested positive for rabies [37], while in 2005, it was shown that male individuals considered to be intruders, with body lesions of up to 90%, would be important in carrying the rabies virus from one group to another and from one region to another [(38).]
- Body lesions, attributed to bites caused by other bats, were found in 76.7% of the *Desmodus* studied, and serology (0.5 IU/ml) showed a 30.1% titre (high viral circulation), despite

this, no individual was positive from the brain samples [(54)].

- It was unpredictable to raise rabies in bats in a space-time dynamic, and treatment with vampiricides did not prevent the anticipation of outbreaks and within the Andean valleys, invasions formed waves that advanced into large populations of unvaccinated cattle, heavily ravaged by bats, increasing transmission and mortality [53].

4. Rabies in herbivores and humans

- The areas where people have died from rabies transmitted by *Desmodus* are undergoing changes in production processes, are in remote areas without adequate medical services and the population is unaware of the risk of transmission via bats, in addition to the fact that houses are very vulnerable to vampire entry [22];
- Human attacks by *Desmodus rotundus* gained great repercussions in 2004 with 21 deaths in Pará and in 2005, 24 in Maranhão. In the first case, mortality in the exposed population was 1.14%, and in the second 1% [23];
- In Argentina, 14 years of studies have shown herbivore outbreaks at a rate of 36 to 40 km per year. When the capture and control of vampires has been studied progressively and in a straight line, the cases sometimes begin to appear on the opposite side, demonstrating that work and vaccination must be carried out in a circular manner [6];
- Rabies outbreaks in herbivores in the Codó Microregion in Maranhão, there has been an increase in rabies of around 95.29 Km^2/year [24]. This reinforces the idea that vampire control must always be at the forefront of the events detected.
- In outbreaks of rabies in herbivores, vaccine boosters in susceptible animals should be carried out within 21 to 30 days, and if there are calves under 3 months of age and their lives are at risk, it's best to vaccinate susceptible animals as soon as possible, as today's vaccines are cell-cultured and don't cause many reactions [1];

5. Control of the Desmodus rotundus or common vampire (vampiricides)

- Control methods must be selective and carried out correctly, in such a way as to only target Desmodus rotundus haematophagous bats [1];
- To use the topical paste, understand that bats spend 2 to 3 hours cleaning themselves every day, put their hind feet in their mouths for 5 to 10 seconds, and clean their wings and

thumbs with their tongues [25];

- The 2% warfarin-based pastes cause internal and subcutaneous haemorrhages in the wings of D. *rotundus*, causing slow movement or difficulty in flying [26], abortions can occur [15], leaving some individuals vulnerable to predators, and before being devoured, they manage to transmit the virus to other susceptible species as a form of defence [5], after treatment with vampiricide pastes, haematophagous wings can be found on the ground [7];
- The capture and treatment of haematophagous bats causes a 90 to 100% reduction in the number of vampires [25]. After treatment on the back of haematophagous bats, there is a low capacity for recovery of the vampire population [6];
- Failures in the use of the paste can occur when bats are released at the end of the night and at dawn, as they tend to look for the first shelters and there are records of them nesting with birds [25];
- The females proved to be more faithful to the shelters and better spreaders of vampiricide paste than the males [27];
- In the case of catches in corrals or food sources, understand that the moon changes every 28 days, with a daily change of 20 minutes. You can also choose to work up to a week after the full moon, but as a precaution the nets in corrals are set at dusk and the work can be finished close to midnight [28];
- The strategy established in the state of São Paulo indicates capturing as many bats as possible in the shelter, with the team working in the same season, returning to the same shelter a year later for evaluation and new control, so they calculate that they capture around 30% more haematophagous bats than the previous year [29];
- The use of pastes around the animals' wounds should be until they stop being harassed for blood, even then, the vampire may choose other animals on the property or attack in neighbouring establishments. If there is too much paste on the wound, the bat may avoid the old bite [5];
- When using paste or pour-on vampiricides, remember that bats return to the same animal in up to 60 per cent of cases [15,30];
- In field conditions, the technique of applying vampiricide paste to cattle wounds for three consecutive days has been shown to be between 81 and 95 per cent effective on several

farms, when the percentage of bite reductions is measured [31];

- A study of cows treated with 2% Warfarin intramuscularly (5mg/kg live weight) and lactating calves indicated that they would have to drink 40 litres of milk in order to ingest 5 mg of the product. Five days after treatment, no residues were found in the tissues that could be harmful for human consumption [0;(3]

4. *Considerations on controlling Desmodus rotundus* [5]

- Successful control depends on factors such as the location of shelters, size and physical space, sexual dimorphism and the number of individuals per colony;
- In more preserved areas, effective control of catches in corrals or shelters can occur in 3 to 5 years or more, due to the movement of bats or even their food source;
- It is wise to contact the owners between 15 and 30 days to assess the success of the treatment;

- When planning *Desmodus* control, consider that the number of bats captured is close to the number of recent bites observed on the animals;
- D. *rotundus* feeds on different sources, with a greater predilection for horses and cattle and a lesser predilection for poultry, but they attack all species at different times;
- In areas such as mangrove swamps, forests, flooded areas or areas that are difficult to access, or shelters are not easily found, so animals can be captured at the source of their food (in corrals) and treated or 'pour on' vampiricides can be used on the injured animals.

7. Paralytic rabies in cattle (RPB)

Rabies is an acute, progressive viral encephalomyelitis that mainly infects carnivores and bats, although any mammal can be affected [42]. It is transmitted through animal-to-animal and animal-to-human bites [43]. Signs in cattle can be anorexia, teeth grinding, apathy, salivation, changes in animal behaviour, mooing, tongue distension, tenesmus, retention of faeces and urine, decreased central and peripheral reflexes, decreased skin sensitivity, staggering gait, progressing to decubitus and subsequent death six to eight days after onset [43,]

[44].

The vampire bat is an important reservoir in Latin America and is the source of several outbreaks in cattle as well as people, particularly in parts of the Amazon. The virus travels via the peripheral nerves to the spinal cord to the brain, then travels back via the peripheral nerves to the salivary glands. The virus is spread intermittently in saliva. Haematogenous spread does not occur. In most cases, there is no danger of aerosol transmission of the rabies virus [42].

The key to controlling zoonoses such as rabies, echinococcosis and brucellosis is to focus on the reservoirs [36]. In the case of herbivore rabies, MAPA recommends vaccinating susceptible animals in outbreak areas and controlling transmitters (the reservoirs are mainly winged animals, almost always Desmodus rotundus), and the Ministry of Agriculture encourages health education for the communities involved. The technical manual on herbivore rabies, version 2009, explains that single male D. rotundus are expelled from the colony and can travel more than 100 kilometres, although their radius of action is less than 15 kilometres.

It has been shown that in 1985, rabies in Africa spread from 30 to 40 kilometres a year, with dogs, jackals and big cats as vectors, and the victims were mainly cattle, humans and antelopes [39]. Studies carried out on foxes by Murray and colleagues in Oxford estimated rabies waves of 6 to 12 years, with dispersals of 200 to 600 km [40]. In Brazil, cycles in wild carnivores (wolves and foxes) have been described as lasting between 3 and 5 years (ZINI, 2005). In Argentina, in 1989, they described cycles of 4 years in herbivores that were transmitted by Desmodus rotundus, and in general, the outbreaks extended just over 100 km^2 in 9 months [(41)]. This also provides epidemiological evidence in a control area for herbivore rabies.

The typical distribution range of D. rotundus activity in an outbreak in RS was approximately 80 km^2, and the outbreak ended suddenly over a period of one month. The affected area was geographically isolated by a valley and a river, which may have limited the bats' activities and distribution by feeding. It is also possible that the size of the Desmodus population in the region is too small to act as a reservoir for the rabies virus. There have also been no outbreaks of rabies there in the last three years, and the outbreak had ended without any specific prevention measures being implemented for rabies in herbivores [45].

In the control of D. rotundus bats and rabies in these vampires, you should consider observing movement in the area, which is covered by a network of interacting colonies, including maternity shelters and male satellites [47].

More recent studies suggest a critical role in the elimination of colonies through the use of vampiricides, often reacting in the form of outbreaks, either through increased movement, due to the release of space in shelters or dispersal mediated by disturbance [48] and death, so the whole epidemiological set must be evaluated in the actions.

In regions with rugged terrain, the work of preventing and controlling rabies and bats could be reduced to just 3 kilometres[58].

A study in Peru from Jul 2007 to Oct 2010, serologies showed that the circulation of the virus in vampires occurred in all years, by captures and repaptures, seroprevalence ranged from 3 to 28% and was higher in juveniles and sub-adults. The vampiricide treatment campaigns implemented during our study failed to reduce seroprevalence due to the removal of adults, since potentially the most important factor was juvenile and sub-adult bats in the transmission of the rabies virus [49].

It should be borne in mind that the detection of antibodies and the Desmodus rabies virus has been known for a long time. The programme (PNCRH) is trying to eliminate viral circulation in susceptible individuals and not in bats, since in rural areas they are the main transmitters. What needs to change is the strategy of treating all individuals who are captured, evaluating occurrences in the area or municipalities where they occur, reporting cases in animals to health personnel, epidemiologically evaluating each situation, alerting and educating communities.

8. *Prevention and control of bovine rabies (Adapted from FAO texts5 and the Manual of the National Programme for the Control of Herbivore Rabies - PNCRH 1):*

The strategy should be formulated on the basis of a periodic risk assessment, review and, if necessary, adjustments to control (try to involve a few municipalities because of the cost of vaccinations to producers), is directed to the Official Veterinary Service (SVO).

Check the risks of diffusion:

The risk of spreading Bovine Paralytic Rabies (BPR), by virus variants, for example 3, by monitoring bats and analysing the occurrence of rabies in the area over time (how many km/year does the virus occur in the area?);

Transmitters: Carnivores - cases are in a straight line (up to 200km/year); Haematophagous bats - cases in circular areas, note that the virus circulates only in the animals that have been attacked, and that horizontal bovine-to-cattle transmission is a myth, as they are the final hosts, still limited to fences;

(Programme strategy: In all circumstances, actions to block the progression of the virus must be carried out from the periphery to the centre of the outbreak. This is because the infected bat can transmit the virus to other colonies up to twelve kilometres away from the initial outbreak or more, depending on the area and the epidemiological assessment).

Check the risks of exposure:

Evaluate the amount of sucking in the susceptible population, herd immunity and active surveillance by the service or passive surveillance by third parties.

Receptivity: the capacity of an ecosystem to harbour populations of Desmodus rotundus (related to the availability of food and shelter).

(Receptivity can be high, medium, low or zero, depending on the presence or interaction of factors such as density of susceptible animal species and pasture formation, % of area with calcareous soil, % of area of permanent forest, number and location of natural and artificial shelters for the vampire and altitude).

Vulnerability: the ability of the transmitter to enter an area and the viral circulation likely to generate new cases in a given area.

Factors that affect vulnerability are the construction of shelters, for example at hydroelectric power stations, roads, railways, as well as deforestation, new areas for grazing, floods, fire and other environmental changes, deaths or abrupt withdrawals from the food source. Observe cases of RPB in neighbouring areas (previous outbreaks) and cases of rabies in other species.

(Vulnerability to Receptivity can be high, medium, low or zero, depending on the presence or interaction of the factors).

In an assessment of the risk of circulation of the rabies virus carried by haematophagous bats (variant 3) in herbivore populations in the Paraíba do Sul River Valley in São Paulo, it was observed that 81.8% of rabies outbreaks were adequately predicted by the model and could have been prevented if strategic vaccination had been adopted in areas at high risk of the virus circulating [50].

9. Guidelines of the National Programme for the Control of Herbivore Rabies - PNCRH[1]

- Registration and monitoring of haematophagous bat shelters;
- Assistance with encephalitis (suspected rabies) and epidemiological investigation of cases;
- Vaccination of domestic herbivores (especially in focal zones and regions epidemiologically considered to be at high risk);
- Control of the haematophagous bat population (D. *rotundus).* In outbreak areas, control of transmitters should be intensified within a radius of 12 kilometres;
- Health education (improving community feedback).

Caring for outbreaks

- The SVO is responsible for carrying out health measures;
- It starts from the moment of the complaint or notification, using the Initial Disease Investigation Form (Form-In);
- The death of the animal occurs on average between 5 and 7 days after the presentation of the signs, from the date of the aggression dogs and cats, or other suspects should be observed for 10 days;

- Handling the carcass of a rabid animal poses a high risk (butchers, handlers, employees, technicians) and also due to consumption by wild animals;
- Closure of the outbreak occurs within 90 days, with the Complementary Disease Investigation Form (Form-Com).

Complaint/Notification (owner, third parties and surveillance)

- Once the complaint has been made, the SVO must verify or reject the occurrence within a period of no more than 24 hours;
- Collect data on species and movements, including periphytosis (number of animals vaccinated against rabies, date of last vaccination, vaccine dose, expiry date, etc.);
- The property will be considered a "suspected nervous disease" until the official veterinarian follows up;
- If the result is positive, contact the health authorities.

Attendance by the Official Veterinary Service (SVO)

- Clinical assessment and epidemiological investigation of the area;
- **Suspected case:** signs compatible with herbivore rabies, plus the presence of animals attacked by haematophagous bats or other transmitters and/or the existence of shelters;
- **Case ruled out:** signs not compatible with herbivore rabies;
- **Compatible diseases:** have clinical signs of encephalitis, which can be poisoning, Aujeszky's disease, cerebral babesiosis, listeriosis, equine encephalitis, among others
- When harvesting the CNS (Central Nervous System), the floor of the cranial cavity should be included, where the trigeminal nerve ganglion (Gasser's ganglion) is located for cases of rabies and Bovine Herpesvirus Meningoencephalitis (BHV-5), and the carotid rete mirabile should be harvested along with the pituitary gland for suspected cases of Malignant Catarrhal Fever [46];

- **Confirmed case or well-founded suspicion:** if the laboratory test is positive, action must be taken on the property involved and neighbouring properties within a 12 km radius considered a Focal Zone, but a 25 km Surveillance Zone must be set up for monitoring (see figure);

- **Distribution of rabies outbreaks by municipality (detail):** Total number of owners; Number of outbreaks per owner; Total number of susceptible animals; Quantities by species affected; Number of MH shelters; Total number of vaccinated animals by species;

- **Distribution of notifications by outbreak area > or = 12 km (detail):** N° of owners;

quantitative by species affected; N° of MH shelters; N° of MH captured and treated in the area; Total N° of animals vaccinated by species;

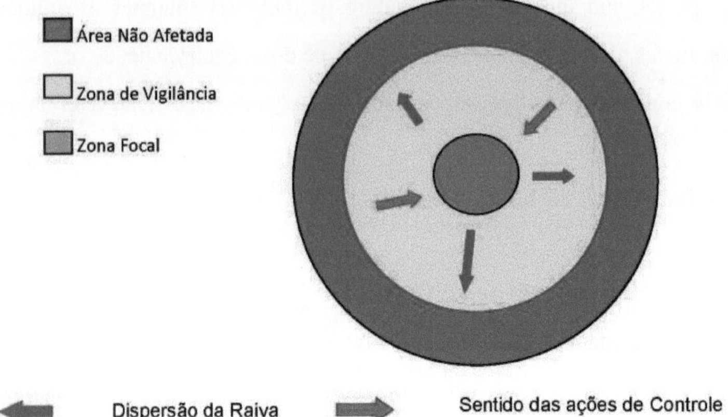

Figure: Model of concentric circles for action in a BPR hotspot. Adapted from: Souza JCP 56, Ministry of Agriculture, Livestock and Supply (MAPA)[1] and Food and Agriculture Organisation of the United Nations (FAO) 57.

Rabies Negatives and the collection of material for BSE testing (Adapted [59])

- For the diagnosis of TSEs in adult ruminants (cattle > 24 months and small ruminants > 12 months of age), the whole brain (entire Central Nervous System) can be sent under refrigeration (2 to 8° C), as long as the sample arrives at the laboratory within 24 hours of collection; if this period exceeds 24 hours, it can be frozen.

- Experiments with *Bovine Spongiform Encephalopathy* in cattle with the *He L type* showed that they all presented the nervous form with some similarities to *classical BSE.* Prominent features were: nervousness, panic when cleaning, apprehension, difficulty getting up, lateral decubitus, drowsiness, disordered walking, which occur naturally in emergency slaughter cattle or when they arrive dead. Both were easily detectable as BSE by current confirmation methods with the obex region, even with the removal of a portion with the spoon through the foramen magnum. The cerebellum proved to be a more reliable sample for indication when using immunohistochemistry.

- ***Notification (by owners/third parties/SVO surveillance):*** the authority informs its headquarters or the other way round, headquarters informs the unit;
- ***Case:*** an animal infected with a pathogen, with or without clinical signs;
- ***Focus:*** one or more cases in an epidemiological unit (group of animals/same space/same pathogen)

Appendix

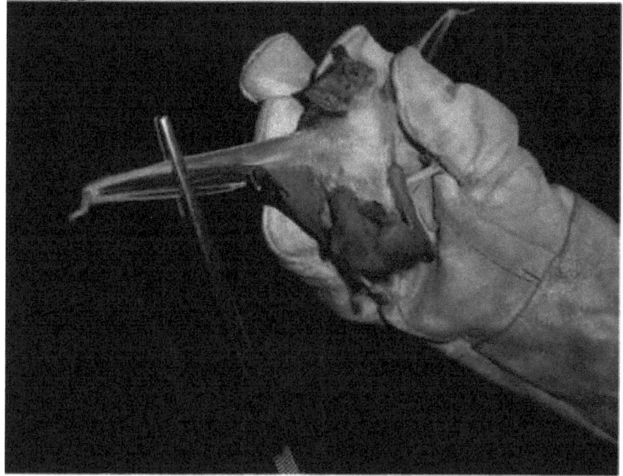

Photo: Detail of the common vampire bat, D. rotundus, with its young. Presidente Figueredo/AM (ARRUDA, 2006).

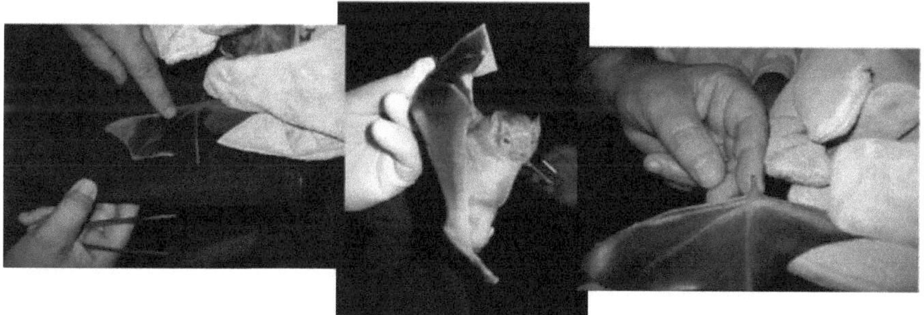

Photo: White-winged vampire bat, *Diaemus youngi,* male with 52mm long right forearm. Raposa/MA (ARRUDA, 2011).

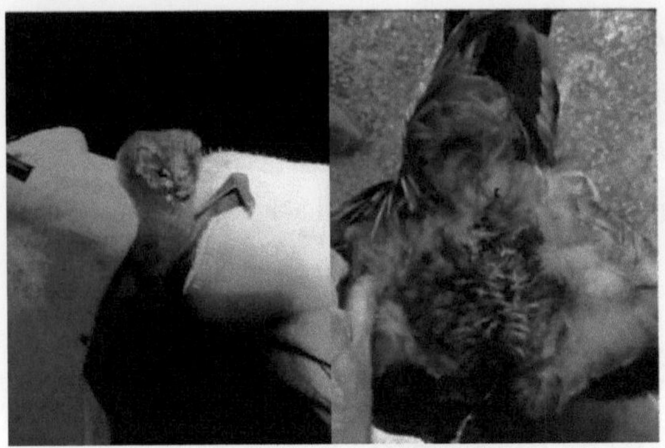

Photo: The hairy-legged vampire bat, Diphylla ecaudata, usually attacks the cloaca of birds. Pesqueira/PE (Pernambuco Agricultural Defence and Inspection Agency / ADAGRO, 2009).

Thank you

To my colleague Angelo Luiz Tadeu Ottati from the Federal Superintendence of Agriculture, Livestock and Supply in the State of Maranhão (SFA-MA- MAPA) for his contribution in formatting the manuscript for this work.

References

1 Brazil, Ministry of Agriculture, Livestock and Supply. Technical Manual. Control of herbivore rabies. Secretariat for Animal Defence. Brasília: DSA. 2009. 124p

2 Wilkinson, G. S. Food Sharing in vampire bat. Scientifc American 1990. 76-82

3 Greenhall, A. M. Etologia y ecologia de los Vampiros... Proceedings ...Consultation meeting on the care of people exposed to vampire rabies. OPS. Washinton, DC. 1991 9p.

4 Flores Crespo R, Limbart SB, Burns RJ, Mitchell GC. J. Mammal 1972. 53;365- 368

5 Arruda RCN, Souza JCP, Barçante JMP, Pereira HM, Santos HP. Evaluation of the control of Desmodus rotundus in forest and mangrove regions of the state of

Maranhão/Brazil. UFLA. 2012. 30p "in press"

[6] Fornes A, Lord RD, Kuns ML, Larghi OP, Fuenzalida E, Lazara L. Control of Bovine rabies through vampire bat control. Journal of Wildlife 1974 Oct; 10:310-316

[7] Costa LM, Esbérard CEL. Desmodus rotundus (Mammalia: Chiroptera), on the south coast of the state of Rio de Janeiro, Brazil. Braz. J. Biol., 2011, 71:(3): 739-746

[8] Rio de Janeiro State Health Department (SES-RJ). Manual for bat management and rabies control. 24p. 2000. Available at: <http://portal.saude.rj.gov.br/Docs/cvas/MANUAL%20DE%20MORCEGO%20ATUSED.pdf>. Accessed 23/07/2010.

[9] Uieda, W. Feeding behaviour of haematophagous bats when attacking poultry, goats and pigs in captive conditions. State University of Campinas. Institute of Biology. Thesis (doctorate). Campinas, SP. 1994.

[10] Greenhall, A.M. Lucha contra los Murcielagos vampiros. Boletin de la Oficina Sanitaria Panamericana 1971 Sep. 232-246

[11] Linhart, S. B. Age determination and occurrence of incremental growth lines in the dental cementum of the common vampire bat (Desmodus rotundus). J. Mammal 1973. 54:493-496

[12] Delpietro HA. Epidemiological situation of herbivore rabies in Argentina. 2001. International Seminar on bats as transmitters of rabies. São Paulo 2001. 76p.

[13] Kiappenbach MA, Murcielagos and vampires. Almanarque del Banco de Seguros del estado. Uruguay 1976. 235-295

[14] Brazil. Ministry of Health. Bats in urban and rural areas: Management and control manual. National Health Foundation 1996. 117p.

[15] Piccinini RS, Peracchi AL, Sousa JCP, Albuquerque ST, Raimundo SDL, Tannure AM, Furtado LL. Behaviour of the haematophagous bat Desmodus rotundus (chiroptera) related to the attack rate on cattle in captivity. Pesq. Vet. Brás. Rio de Janeiro. 1985. 5(4):111-116.

[16] Cabeza de Vaca A.N. 2009. Naufrágios e comentários (Translation by Jurandir Soares dos Santos). 2ª ed. L&PM, Porto Alegre. 240p.

[17] Scheffer, Karin Corrêa et al. Rabies virus in naturally infected chiroptera in the State of São Paulo, Brazil. Rev. Saúde Pública [online]. 2007, vol. 41, no. 3, pp. 389-395. ISSN 0034-8910.

[18] Sodré, M. M.; Gama, A. R. da; Almeida, M. F. de. Updated list of bat species positive for rabies in Brazil. Rev. Inst. Med. Trop. Sao Paulo 2010, March-April. 52 (2):75-81,

[19] Arruda, R. C. N. de. Rabies and encephalitis in domestic herbivores in the state of Maranhão: diagnosis, georeferencing and proposed technique for brain collection in bats. 2011. 71f Dissertation (Master's in Animal Science) - State University of Maranhão, São Luís, 2011.

[20] Silva JA, Moreira EC, Haddad JPA, Modena CM, Tubaldini MAS. Temporal and special distribution of rabies in Minas Gerais, 1976 to 1997. Arq. Bras. Med. Vet. Zootec., v.55, n.3, 2001,p.680 to 684.

[21] Silva RC, Langoni H, Menozzi BD, Camossi LG, Greca Junior HG, Camargo LB, Faccioli PY. Maintenance of rabies virus in non-hematophagous bats (Artibeus lituratus and Myotis spp.) in Botucatu, SP. Biological, São Paulo 2006: 68;140-142

[22] Schneider MC, Santos-Burgoa C S. Algunas consideraciones sobre la rabia humana transmitida por murciélago. Salud Pública de México 1995. 37:354-362.

[23] Schneider MC, Romijn PC, Uieda W, Tamayo H, Da Silva DF, Belotto A, Da Silva JB, Leanes LF. Rabies transmitted by vampire bats tohumans: An emerging zoonotic disease in Latin America? Rev Panam Salud Publica/Pan Am J Public Health 2009; 25(3)

[24] Arruda RCN, Sena EF, Costa FN, Santos HP, Pereira HM, Monte SS, Campos H, Waquim SJ, Batista H B CR. Retrospective and spatial study of rabies in herbivores in the microregion of Codo/Maranhão - Brazil. XX Meeting International the Rabies of America (RITA) Québec - Canada 2009, Oct 18 to 23.

[25] Linhart SB, Flores Crespo R, Mitchell GC. Control of vampire bats by topical application of an anticoagulant, Chlorophacinone. Bol. Ofic. Sanit. Panamer 1972. 6:31-38.

[26] Pozetti, P. S. Control of haematophagous bats by spraying 2% technical warfarin on horses in captivity. 59f. Dissertation (Master's Degree in Preventive Veterinary Medicine) - Federal Rural University of Rio de Janeiro. Rio de Janeiro. 1993.

[27] Gomes, M. N.; Uieda, W. Diurnal shelters, colony composition, sexual dimorphism and reproduction of the haematophagous bat D. rotundus (E. Geoffroy). [Chiroptera, Phyllostomidae] in the state of São Paulo, Brazil. Revista Brasileira de Zoologia. 21 (3) p 629-638, 2004.

[28] Flores Crespo R. Tecnicas, substancias y estrategia s para el control de murcielagos vampiros. Pan American Health Organisation. 2003 Mar. 12p.

[29] Pasteur Institute. Manual for the control of herbivore rabies. Pasteur Institute, São Paulo 2010. 58p.

[30] Flores Crespo R. Techniques to control vampire bats. Epidemiologist Ministry of Heath, Lima Peru 1990 p.19-29

[31] Flores-Crespo R. Biología y control de murciélagos vampiros. En: Rabia en las diferentes especies, sus transmisores y su control. pp 93-94. Ed R Flores-Crespo 1998.

[32] Lord RD, Muradali F, Lazaro I. Age composition of vampire bats (Desmodus rotundus) in Northern Argentina and Southern Brazil . J. Mammalogy 1976, 57:573- 575.

[33] Delpietro H, Diaz AMO, Fuenzalida E, Bell JF. Determining the rabies attack rate in murcielagos. Bol. Of. San. Pan 1972. 63:222-230.

[34] Lord RD, Fuenzalida E, Delpietro H, Larghi OP, Diaz AMO, Lazaro L. Observations on the epizootiology of vampire bat rabies. Bull. Pan. Am. Health Org. 1975.9:189-195.

[35] Lord RD. An ecological strategy for controlling bovine rabies through elimination of vampire bats. Proceedings of the 9th Vertebrate Pest Conference, 1980. 169-175

[36] Zinsstag J, Schelling E, Roth F, Bonfoh B, De Savigny D, Tanner M. Human benefits of animal interventions for zoonosis control. Important rabies references. Emerg Infect Dis. 2007 Apr;13(4):527-31.

[37] Côrtes, V.A., Souza, l.C., Uieda, W. & Figuereido, a.c. 1994. Daytime shelters and rabies infection in bats from Botucatu, São Paulo, Brazil. Veterinária e Zootecnia, São Paulo, 6: 179-186.

[38] Rocha, fabrícia aparecida da. Diurnal Shelters, Groupings and Body Injuries in the Haematophagous Bat Desmodus rotundus (Chiroptera, Phyllostomidae) from the

(Master's Degree in Veterinary Medicine). São Paulo State University. Botucatu, SP. 2005.

[39] Kuwert, E. Merieux, C. Koprowski, H. Konrad Bogel. Rabies in the Tropics. Spring-Verlag. Berlin. Heidelberg. New York. Tokyo. 1985.

[40] Cliff, A. Haggett, P. Smallman-Raynor, M. World Atlas of Epidemic Diseases. 2004.

[41] Delpietro HA. Nader AJ. Rabies of herbivores transmitted by vampire bats in north-eastern Argentina. 1989

[42] The Merck Veterinary Manual. Overview of Rabies. Available at: http://www.merckvetmanual.com/mvm/nervous_system/rabies/overview_of_rabies.h tml. Accessed on 07 Mar. 2016.

[43] Aytekin I. Mamak N. A Case of Rabies in a Cow. Journal of Animal and Veterinary Advances. 2009. 8 (12):2760-2762.

[44] REIS, M. C., COSTA, J. N., PEIXOTO, A.P.C., FIGUEIREDO, L. J. C., MENEZES, R. V., FERREIRA, M. M., SÁ, J. E. U. Clinical and epidemiological aspects of bovine rabies presented in the casuistry of the Bovine Clinic (Oliveira dos Campinhos, Santo Amaro, Bahia), Federal University of Bahia, during the period from January 1990 to December 1999 (Case report). Rev. Bras. Saúde Prod. An., v.4, n.1, p. 12-17, 2003.

[45] Itou T , Fukayama T, Mochizuki N , Kobayashi Y, Deberaldini ER, Carvalho AAB, Ito FH, Sakai T. Molecular epidemiological tracing of a cattle rabies outbreak lasting less than a month in Rio Grande do Sul in southern Brazil. Available at:

http://bmcresnotes.biomedcentral.com/articles/10.1186/s13104-016-1898-5. Accessed 07 Mar. 2016.

[46] Brazil, Ministry of Agriculture, Livestock and Supply. Procedures for the diagnosis of central nervous system diseases in cattle / Claudio Severo Lombardo Barros and Guilherme

Henrique Figueiredo Marques. Brasília : MAPA/SDA/DDA, 2003. 50 p.

[47] Johnson N, Aréchiga-Ceballos N and Aguilar-Setien A. Vampire Bat Rabies: Ecology, Epidemiology and Control. Viruses 2014, 6, 1911-1928. Available at: http://www.ncbi.nlm.nih.gov/pmc/articles/PMC4036541/pdf/viruses-06-01911.pdf. Accessed 08 Mar. 2016.

[48] Blackwood, J.C.; Streicker, D.G.; Altizer, D.; Rohani, P. Resolving the roles of immunity, pathogenesis, and immigration for rabies persistence in vampire bats. *Proc. Natl. Acad. Sci. USA* 2013, 110, 20837-20842.

[49] Streicker DG, Recuenco S, Valderrama W, Benavides JG, Vargas I, Pacheco V, Condori REC, Montgomery J, Rupprecht CE, Rohani P and Altizer S. Ecological and anthropogenic drivers of rabies exposure in vampire bats: implications for transmission and control. Proc. R. Soc. B. 2012. Available at: http://rspb.royalsocietypublishing.org/content/royprsb/279/1742/3384.full.pdf. Accessed on 09 Mar. 2016.

[50] Dias RA, Nogueira Filho VS, Goulart CS, Telles ICO, Marques GHF, Ferreira F, et al. Risk model for rabies virus circulation in herbivores in the State of São Paulo, Brazil. Rev Panam Salud Publica. 2011;30(4):370-6.

[51] Trajano E. Movements of Cave Bats in Southeastern Brazil, with Emphasis on the Population Ecology of the Common Vampire Bat, Desmodus rotundus (Chiroptera). Biotropica, Vol. 28, No. 1 (Mar., 1996), pp. 121-129.

[52] Theimer TC, Dyer AC, Keeley BW, Gilbert AT, Bergman DL. Ecological Potential for Rabies Virus Transmission via Scavenging of Dead Bats by Mesocarnivores. Journal of Wildlife Diseases 2017 53 (2), 382-385.

[53] Benavides JA, Valderrama W, Streicker DG. 2016 Spatial expansions and travelling

waves of rabies in vampire bats. Proc. R. Soc. B 283: 20160328. Available at: ftp://dx.doi.org/10.1098/rspb.2016.0328. Accessed on 02 May 2017.

[54] Ferrari , JJF & Marrelli, Mt. Common haematophagous bat Desmodus rotundus in the Paraíba Valley, São Paulo State: diurnal shelters, groupings, body lesions and anti-rabies serology (2015). Available at: <www.teses.usp.br/teses/disponiveis/6/6132/tde-03082015-113130/ > 02 May 17.

[55] Streicker DG, Recuenco S, Valderrama W, Gomez Benavides J, Vargas I, Pacheco V, Condori Condori RE, Montgomery J, Rupprecht CE, Rohani P, Altizer S. Ecological and anthropogenic drivers of rabies exposure in vampire bats: implications for transmission and control. Available at: <https://www.ncbi.nlm.nih.gov/pubmed/22696521>. 02 May. 17.

[56] Souza JCP: Control of haematophagous bats Population dynamics. Course on the control of wild rabies (D. rotundus) in Brazil. Veterinary Public Health Unit. Pan American Foot and Mouth Disease Centre. Rio de Janeiro. p.17-20. 2007. Available at: < http://ww3.panaftosa.org.br/Comp/MAPA/29314.pdf>. 26 Jan 17.

[57] United Nations Food and Agriculture Organisation (FAO). Course: Rabies of herbivores and "One Health"... Moving towards integrated health management. Bovine Rabies Prevention and Control Programmes. Unit - 6 Vampiricide. Available at: http://www.fao.org/in-action/capacitacion-politicas- publicas/cursos/ver/en/c/294538/>. 02 May 17.

[58] Puga, LCHP. Spatial modelling of the occurrence of haematophagous bat bites in the Zona da Mata of Minas Gerais. 2015. 104 f. Thesis (Doctorate in Veterinary Medicine). Federal University of Viçosa. Minas Gerais. 2015. Available at: <http://www.locus.ufv.br/bitstream/handle/123456789/6746/texto%20com pleto.pdf?sequence=1>. Accessed 26 Jan 17.

[59] Brazil. Ministry of Agriculture, Livestock and Supply. Brazilian Bovine Spongiform

Encephalopathy (BSE) Prevention and Surveillance System. DSA/MAPA. Brasília. 15p. April 2014

Encephalopathy (BSE) Prevention and Surveillance System. DSA/MAPA. Brasília. 15p. April 2014

CHAPTER 2

REPORT: HOW TO PREVENT CHIROPTERA IN RURAL ESTABLISHMENTS BY USING MOSQUITO NETTING ON THE EAVES

Roberto Carlos Negreiros de Arruda [1]

Éric Takashi Kamakura de Carvalho Mesquita [2]

Karlos Yuri Fernandes Pedrosa [2]

Summary

Bat refuges in rural homes are a constant problem when the establishments are not continuously inhabited. People are afraid to live or sleep in a rural home because of bat flights, as well as the aggravation of coming into contact with faeces on the walls and floor, and/or accidental contact with bats. The aim of this report was to demonstrate the installation of mosquito screens around the eaves of a rural home, using simple and affordable materials, even in rural areas. The screen is installed by attaching the flat wire to the rafters and laths in such a way as to fix the upper part to the roof, as well as fixing the lower part of the screen with a channel, leaving no escape area, thus avoiding the entry of permanent bats, as well as mitigating the risk of a relationship that could spread diseases, such as rabies or contact with faeces, to people with sensitive skin, or debilitated people prone to lung problems due to histoplasmosis. The result of this manual labour was to promote greater leisure for residents and visitors to the rural property, and we also believe that these screens extended to the doors and windows hinder the transmission of diseases such as dengue, zika, chikungunya and yellow fever, preventing mosquitoes from entering and biting.

Keywords: Bats, colonies, shelters, abandoned houses and mosquito netting.

[1] Master in Animal Science and Federal Agricultural Tax Auditor for the Ministry of Agriculture, Livestock and Supply (MAPA).

São Luís/MA. Author for correspondence: rcnegreiros.arruda@gmail.com

[2] State Agricultural Inspector of the Maranhão State Agricultural Defence Agency (AGED/MA)

Introduction

Bat refuges in rural dwellings are a constant problem when there is no permanent dwelling place for people, or when rural establishments are not inhabited continuously, as well as when the visual relationship between people and colonies, or even the noise or odour, is a nuisance.

The aim of this report was to present a model for installing mosquito netting around a rural establishment to contain non-hematophagous or haematophagous bats, avoiding human contact with the bats, since such contact can spread diseases such as rabies and histoplasmosis.

Report

We were asked to give our opinion on a way of controlling bats in rural homes in a non-aggressive, economical and permanent way, in other words, a solution to an old problem, because many people were afraid to sleep because of the night flights of bats, as well as the aggravation of coming into contact with faeces, either on the walls or on the floor, or even accidental contact with bats.We opted to use mosquito netting to prevent the bats from returning to their former refuges or shelters, without causing any disturbance to the colonies, people or domestic animals, even if it's just nearby, as there are other residences on farms with plenty of fruit and insects. Non-haematophagous bat droppings were found on the walls (Photo 1) and on the ceramic floor of the establishment, as there was a cluster in the bathroom and another in one of the bedrooms.

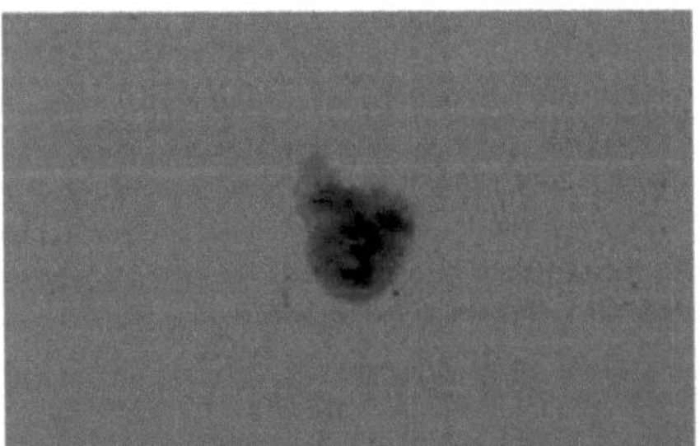

Photo 1: Non-hematophagous bat faeces on the wall.

For a better understanding, the eaves are the final part of the roof, which is made up of a wooden structure, assembled by rafters and slats to which the roof tiles are attached. The eaves serve to deflect rain, and are 0.80cm from the walls externally, and are not always sealed, in which case they form empty spaces between the roof and the wall, allowing bats to roost, enter and exit.

There was no roof over the house, but it was necessary to seal off access to the roof for individuals, as they used the space as a breeding shelter and as a digestive shelter (when feeding at night). The rural residence was used occasionally, on holidays and weekends, located in the municipality of São José de Ribamar, in the state of Maranhão.

The installation was carried out using simple materials that were easy to buy or easily found in rural areas (see table of materials).

The mesh was installed by attaching the flat wire to the rafters and slats in such a way as to fix the upper part of the mesh to the roof, leaving no escape area for the chiroptera, taking care to twist the mesh into a triangular shape when fixing the parts with the channel, thus avoiding pockets or even undesirable cuts in the process (Photo 2). Two screws with dowels were used per channel, every 10 cm from the end of the channel.

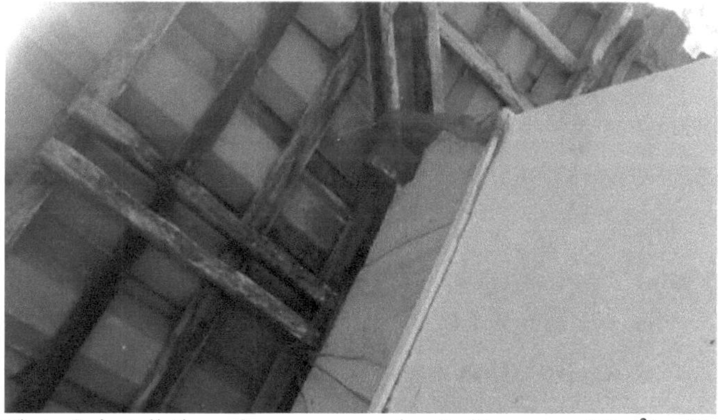

Photo 2: installation of eaves screens in a built-up area ($56m^2$) with profile pvc ducting for the electricity network.

We tried to work on installing screens during the day to scare bats away from their family agglomerations (clusters). The work was carried out over two days.

As a result, the groupings of bats were broken up, moving away to undefined locations, and to date there have been no reports of the colonies returning.

Residents and visitors are therefore encouraged to enjoy themselves more by avoiding contact between chiropters and humans or domestic animals, such as domestic cats *(Felis catus),* which are skilful predators.

Table. List of materials purchased, quantities, market prices and daily rates for the service of installing the screens around the house

Description	Quantity	R$ Unit Value	R$ Value Subtotal
Green mosquito screen 10m long by 1.50m wide	10	4,80	40,80
White PVC channel Partition 20x10x2000mm	13	2,39	31,00
Screws with S-6 Phill bush 6mm	50	0,90	4,50
Smooth galvanised (annealed) wire No. 12. 1 kg roll	1	25,00	25,00
Professionals in 2 days of service	2	180,00	360,00
		R$ Total Value	461,30

Source: João Luiz de Carvalho

Discussion

Humans have shared buildings with bats for thousands of years, probably when the first humans built their primitive huts (VOIGT et al, 2016b), but this coexistence is not well accepted by modern society today.

Humans have inadvertently modified the global ecosystems of bats, and some organisms can tolerate human activities and even flourish in anthropogenic habitats (VOIGT et al, 2016a), with some adjustments to the screens between the wall and eaves we can avoid them, or force them to move to another refuge.

We believe that the bats have moved to shelter in nearby areas, as there are many fruit trees in other neighbouring farms, for example, Bernard & Fenton, studying bat mobility in forests and savannas in Pará in 2003, by marking, recapture and radio telemetry, state that they generally cover distances of 0.5 to 2.5 km from the shelters.

The presence of bats in buildings, especially insectivores, can cause faeces to accumulate, causing unpleasant and characteristic odours. These accumulations can also attract coprophagous insects (Brasil, 1998). In our case, there was no accumulation due to the cleaning carried out.

Humans can develop histoplasmosis after inhaling microscopic spores of *Histoplasma capsulatum* in a heavily contaminated environment. However, cases are rarely fatal, but infections in individuals with weakened immune systems can become serious (MARTINS et al, 2000).

From a list of rabies-positive bat species in Brazil from 1996 to 2009, it comprised 41 international and national species, belonging to 25 genera and three families: Phyllostomidae 43.9%, Vespertilionidae 29.3% and Molossidae 26.8% (SODRÉ, 2010). The presence of rabies virus in the colonies removed for our report was not assessed.

It has been suggested that bat faeces have antigenic properties, causing skin rashes in susceptible humans (Alonso et al., 1998). Cases in which humans have been bitten by the common vampire bat, *Desmodus rotundus*, have been increasing in Brazil. In addition to causing losses by feeding on bovine blood and being a vector for the rabies virus, bats have become a target for control activities by communities and governments (MAYEN, 2003).

Not surprisingly, farmers and ranchers with economic losses caused by bats are more likely to have negative attitudes or report a desire to destroy bat refuges (REID, 2013), diverging from our thinking and direction in carrying out the service in rural establishments.

Although many aromatic compounds and chemical irritants have been proposed and tested as bat repellents, their effectiveness has been very limited, and prolonged inhalation of naphthalene vapours can be dangerous to human health, and the results of using ultrasound have not been promising, while lighting has proved to be more effective (CWDM, 2005). The house already used light-coloured roof tiles among other clay tiles and even left electric lights on at night, without solving the problem.

Some bats live in buildings, and there is no reason to drive them out if there is little chance of contact with people. To prevent them from entering, close up large openings in the home, use screens on windows, doors or chimney caps, in attics or belvederes, fill electrical and plumbing holes with stainless steel wool or seal. Watch where the bats come out at dusk and keep clear plastic or bird netting over these areas. The bats may even crawl out, but they can't come back in. When all the bats are gone, the openings can be permanently sealed (CDC, 2016). Another procedure that can be adopted is to adapt a "bat escape system" at the exit of the shelter, which can be made from PVC pipes and plastic tarpaulins that are cheap and easy to handle (CEVS/RS, 2012). Unlike our mosquito net assembly, these methods are used in small areas, not in an entire rural home.

Bats are rarely aggressive, even when chased, but they can bite in self-defence when grabbed, as with all wild animals, so they should never be handled with bare hands (BCI, 2016). Any type of capture should be carried out by trained and vaccinated personnel.

PAEZ et al, 2008, identified an outbreak of rabies in humans in Colombia, originating from the vampire bat, D. rotundus, whose transmitter was a cat, which confirms the link between domestic species and rabies of wild origin in an urban ecosystem.

This report opens up new perspectives for the continuous installation of a screen around the eaves of a building, preventing the reintroduction of haematophagous or non-hematophagous bats into rural establishments. In addition, the cost of control on the rural property was relatively low, less than R$500.00 ($158.63), without harming the winged creatures or exposing them to natural predators in urban environments.

References

ALONSO A, IRANETA SG, RODRÍGUEZ SM, SCAVINI LM, RODRÍGUEZ SR (1998). **Bat faeces as an indoor allergen.** J Investig Allergol Clin Immunol 8:365- 369.

BERNARD E. FENTON MB. **Bat Mobility and Roosts in a Fragmented Landscape in Central Amazonia, Brazil'**. Biotropica. Volume 35, Issue 2, pages 262-277, June 2003 Available in: < http://onlinelibrary.wiley.com/doi/10.1111/j.1744-7429.2003.tb00285.x/abstract>. Accessed on 05 January 2016.

BCI. BAT CONSERVATION INTERNATIONAL. **Excluding bate from buildings.** USA. 2016. Available at:< http://www.batcon.org/index.php/resources/for-specific-issues/bats-in-buildings>. Accessed on 07 January 2016.

BRAZIL. MINISTRY OF HEALTH. **Bats in urban and rural areas - management and control manual. Brasilia.** Bredt et al (eds), Fundação Nacional

Health. 1998. 117p. Available at:< http://docslide.com.br/documents/morcegos- em-areas-urbanas-e-rurais-manual-de-manejo-e-controle.html>. 07 Jan. 2016.

CDC. CENTRES FOR DISEASE CONTROL AND PREVENTION. **Keeping bats out of your house.** USA. 2016. Available at:< http://www.cdc.gov/rabies/bats/management/>. Accessed on 07 Jan. 2016.

CWDM. CENTRE FOR WILDLIFE DAMAGE MANAGEMENT. **Bats**. USA. 2005. Available at:< http://icwdm.org/handbook/mammals/bats.asp>. Accessed on 07 January 2016.

CEVS/RS. STATE HEALTH SURVEILLANCE CENTRE. GOVERNMENT OF THE STATE OF RIO GRANDE DO SUL. **Guide to bat management and control: identification, capture and collection techniques.** Porto Alegre: CEVS/RS, 2012. Available in: <http://www.saude.rs.gov.br/upload/1350310970_Guia%20de%20Campo%20Morce gos.pdf >. Accessed on 07 January 2016.

MARTINS P, NEVES C, LOPES AA, SANTOS Q, ARAÚJO NN, PEREIRA M (2000). **Histoplasmosis presenting as acute respiratory distress syndrome after exposure to bat faeces in a home.** Braz J Infect Dis 4:103-106. Available at:< http://europepmc.org/abstract/med/10797657>. 05 Jan. 2016.

MAYEN F (2003) **Haematophagous bats in Brazil, their role in rabies transmission, impact on public health, livestock industry and alternatives to an indiscriminate reduction of bat population.** J Vet Med B Infect Dis Vet Public Health*50:469^472.*

Available in: <http://www.readcube.com/articles/10.1046%2Fj.1439-0450.2003.00713.x?r3_referer=wol&tracking_action=preview_click&show_checkout=1&purchase_referrer=onlinelibrary.wiley.com&purchase_site_license=LICENSE_DENIED>. Accessed on 05 January 2016.

PAEZ A, POLO L, HEREDIA D, NUNEZ C, RODRIGUEZ M, AGUDELO C, PARRA E, PAREDES A, MORENO T y REY G. Outbreak of cat-borne human rabies in the municipality of Santander de Quilichao, Colombia. Revista de Salud Pública - Volumen 11(6), Diciembre 2009. Available at:< http://www.scielosp.org/pdf/rsap/v11n6/v11n6a09.pdf>. Accessed on 10 January 2016.

REID JL. **Restoring birds, bats, and dispersal mutualisms in a tropical agricultural landscape.** University of California, Santa Cruz. 2013.

SODRÉ MM, GAMA A R, ALMEIDA MF. **Updated list of bat species positive for rabies in Brazil.** Rev. Inst. Med. Trop. Sao Paulo. 52(2):75-81, March-April, *2010.* Available at:< *www.revistas.usp.br/rimtsp/article/download/31306/33191>.* Accessed on 10 January 2016.

VOIGT CC. KINGSTON T. **Bats in the Anthropocene: Conservation of Bats in a Changing World.** Spring open. ISBN 978-3-319-25220-9 (eBook). 601p. 2016a.

VOIGT CC. PHELPS KL. AGUIRRE LF. SCHOEMAN MC. VANITHARANI J & ZUBAID, A. Bats and Buildings: The Conservation of Synanthropic Bats. In: Voigt, C.C. and Kingston, T. (eds.), **Bats in the Anthropocene: Conservation of Bats in a Changing World.** DOI 10.1007/978-3-319-25220-9_14. Chapter 14. 2016b. p. 427-462.

CHAPTER 3

OUTBREAKS OF BOVINE RABIES AND THE CARAJÁS RAILWAY IN MARANHÃO

Roberto Carlos Negreiros de Arruda[1],

Anizio José Rocha[2]

Summary

With the initial aim of assessing the impact of the construction of the Estreito Hydroelectric Power Plant and the displacement of Desmodus rotundus on rabies cases in the western region of the state of Maranhão, from 2007 to 2013, Quantum GIS software specialising in mapping was used as a method of spatial analysis. The evaluation shows that the outbreaks of rabies in the Tocantins region are close to Açailândia, and follow the Carajás Railway at least 45 kilometres per year. Of the 16 cases observed, 90% are in the municipality of Açailândia itself. Attention is drawn to the highways and the North-South Railway, which require greater surveillance, capture and treatment of Desmodus rotundus, as new cases could occur. We conclude that the construction of the Estreito Hydroelectric Power Station has displaced haematophagous bats with rabies virus to other locations, but has not spread much to nearby foci, or in the municipalities bordering it (the probable site of spread), however those sick bats that have taken shelter on the Carajás Railway have caused a real negative impact on cattle farming in the region.

Key words: Hydroelectric Power Plant, Railways, Desmodus rotundus and Herbivores

[1] Federal Agricultural Inspector of the Ministry of Agriculture, Livestock and Food Supply (Maranhão/Brazil)

[2] Maranhão State Agricultural Defence Agency - AGED/MA (Maranhão/Brazil)

Background

The hypothesis that haematophagous bats Desmodus rotundus are the transmitters of rabies was proposed in Brazil in 1911 by Carini.

Rabies is transmitted through the penetration of the virus contained in the saliva of the infected animal, mainly by biting and, more rarely, by scratching and licking mucous membranes or open wounds (Brasil, 2005), so many people know that rabies is not transmitted between herbivore herds through blood or when D. rotundus feed.

To recognise the shelters of Desmodus bats, you should look for dark, slimy droppings with an ammoniacal smell (Greenhall, 1991)

The findings show that the first turbine at the Estreito Hydroelectric Power Station in Maranhão was switched on at the end of 2010, but was not yet operating at full capacity.

The Carajás Railway, a railway specialising in the transport of minerals, runs for 892 km from the Serra dos Carajás mines in Parauapebas in the state of Pará to São Luís, the capital of Maranhão, passing through the Toncatina region. It was inaugurated in 1985.

The Carajás Railway did not have regular cases of rabies in herbivores along its route, and as a result did not undergo a continuous process of capturing and treating Desmodus.

Cases of rabies near the Açailândia region increased a lot in 2013, and some properties with cases of rabies were left without a laboratory diagnosis, but it is estimated that around 900 animals died, most of them cattle, but equines also died of rabies on properties in that region.

The aim of our survey was to verify the impact of the construction of the hydroelectric power station on the displacement of haematophagous bats and the appearance of rabies outbreaks in the Tocantins region.

Material and methods

An assessment was made of rabies cases in the western region of the state of Maranhão, from 2007 to 2013, using outbreak mapping and the Quantum GIS programme, which is technical software for studying populations and their spatial geography.

Results and discussions

Evaluating the impact of the Estreito Hydroelectric Power Station, when it closed the floodgate, it filled the shelters, caves and hiding places of the haematophagous bats, and with this they moved to Açailândia and new cases of rabies in the western region of the state of Maranhão, with a larger cattle herd.

In Minas Gerais, the occurrence of rabies in cattle from 1976 to 2004 was evaluated in the municipalities of Aimorés, Ituela and Resplendor, in relation to the area of impact of the Aimorés Hydroelectric Power Plant, corresponding to a radius of 31 km^2, the bovine effect tripled in three decades and at the time it was predicted that there would be no significant impact on the occurrence of a rabies epidemic (LISE, 2006). In our case, the Estreito Hydroelectric Power Station is located on the Tocantins River. On the Maranhão side, it is 200 kilometres from Açailandia/MA, where most of the outbreaks have occurred, and has not spread much to the municipalities bordering Estreito/MA.

We found that the outbreaks of rabies in the Açailândia region are close to the Carajás Railway (Figure 1), since the train leaves Carajás in Pará and heads for Maranhão with a sequence of outbreaks, Cidelândia (1), Açailândia (10), Bom Jesus das Selvas (1), Buriticupu (1), Alto Alegre do Pindaré (0), Santa Inês (0), Vitória do Mearim (0), Santa Rita (0) and São Luís in Maranhão (1), all with cases of rabies in the Tocantins region.

Of the four (4) municipalities through which the railway passes, 16 outbreaks were observed, of which 62.5 per cent were in the municipality of Açailândia, as well as the others in Bom Jesus das Selvas (1) and Itinga (3), all within 40 km of the Carajás Railway.

The first outbreak of 2013 in Açailândia was in the village of Novo Bacabal, originating from a herd of Murrah buffalo (Bubalus bubalis Linnaeus, 1758) from the Baixada Maranhense. In this case, the laboratory test confirmed Variant 3 linked to D. rotundus.

The cohabitation of D. rotundus with other bat species favours rabies endemism (Silva et al, 2001). Artibeus (fruit-eating) and Myotis (insect-eating) have been observed with the same variant 3 as Desmodus rotundus (Silva et al, 2006), and in the area of our studies, other species may help in the dynamism of rabies in the Tocantins region.

Of the outbreaks in Açailândia, the highest incidence was in 2013 (90%), but apparently this was not shown to be directly related to the start of the hydroelectric dam, since considering the distance in a straight line, the municipality would be 180 km from it, but indirectly, if we consider that each year, it is observed that the cases advance at least 45 km, due to the displacement of winged transmitters, by artificial shelters on roads and railways (figure 2).

In the state of Maranhão, rabies outbreaks in herbivores in the Codó Microregion were found to be spreading at a rate of 95.29 Km^2/year (Arruda et al, 2009), reinforcing the idea that vampire control must always be at the forefront of the events detected.

In Argentina, 14 years of studies have shown herbivore outbreaks at a rate of 36 to 40 kilometres per year. When vampire captures and control were studied progressively and in a straight line, the cases sometimes began to appear on the opposite side, demonstrating that work and vaccination should be carried out in a circular fashion (Fornes et al, 1974). In the case of railway lines, D. rotundus capture and control should be carried out in both directions of the line (figures 3 and 4).

The outbreaks are being linked to sick haematophagous bats that are using the Carajás Railway as a shelter, so as a preventative measure they are carrying out a compulsory vaccination of herds in that region, and the measures are being explained in leaflets distributed to producers, as well as the capture and treatment of Desmodus.

In Argentina, as in other areas where bats live, shelters are visited by carnivorous predators to feed on dead or fallen bats. The renewal rate of shelters has been 4 years, with no record of rabies (Delpietro, 2001).

In outbreaks of rabies in herbivores, vaccine boosters for susceptible animals should be carried out within 21 to 30 days for those that have been vaccinated in the first place (Brazil, 2009).

In the Imperatriz Regional Unit, on the banks of the North-South Railway, which crosses through the city of Estreito, there were few cases. In São Francisco do Brejão, a dairy region on the railway, no cases were found, but they should also be worked on. It should be noted that the municipality of Açailândia is at the crossroads of these railways (Carajás/Norte Sul), increasing the chances of cases being directed towards the Norte Sul railway.

Conclusion

The construction of the Estreito Hydroelectric Power Station displaced haematophagous bats with rabies virus to other locations, but did not spread many outbreaks to the municipalities bordering the municipality of Estreito/MA. However, the sick bats that took shelter on the Carajás Railway had a real impact on cattle farming in the region, especially in the municipality of Açailândia.

Reference

ARRUDA RCN, SENA EF, COSTA FN, SANTOS HP, PEREIRA HM, MONTE SS, CAMPOS H, WAQUIM SJ, BATISTA H B CR. **Retrospective and spatial study of rabies in herbivores in the microregion of Codo/Maranhão -** *BRAZILX* XX Meeting International the Rabies of America (RITA) Québec - Canada 2009, Oct 18 a 23.

BRAZIL. Ministry of Agriculture, Livestock and Supply. **Technical Manual. Control of herbivore rabies.** Secretariat for Animal Defence. Brasília: DSA. 2009. 124p

BRAZIL. Ministry of Health. **Epidemiological Surveillance Guide.** Health Surveillance Secretariat. Brasília: Ministry of Health; 2005.

CARINI A. **Sur une grande épizootic de rage.** Ann Inst Pasteur 1911;25:843- 6.

DELPIETRO HA. **Epidemiological situation of herbivore rabies in Argentina. 2001.** International Seminar on bats as transmitters of rabies. São Paulo 2001. 76p

FORNES A, LORD RD, KUNS ML, LARGHI OP, FUENZALIDA E, LAZARA L. **Control of Bovine rabies through vampire bat control.** Journal of Wildlife 1974 Oct; 10:310-316

GREENHALL, A. M. **Etologia y ecologia de los Vampiros.** ...Anais ...Reunion de consulta sobre la attencion a personas expuestas a la rabia transmitida por vampiros. OPS. Washinton, DC. 1991 9p.

LISE, Michael Laurence Zini. **Bovine rabies in the impact area of the Aimorés hydroelectric dam, Minas Gerais, Brazil.** 2005. 46 f.

Dissertation (Master's Degree in Epidemiology) - Postgraduate Programme at the Veterinary School of the Federal University of Minas Gerais, Belo Horizonte, 2005. Available at: <http://www.bibliotecadigital.ufmg.br/dspace/handle/1843/BUOS- 8C5GEN>. Accessed 20/09/2016.

QGIS. QUANTUM GIS. QGIS 2.8.2. Version 2.10.1. Available at <http://qgis.org/en/site/>. Accessed 04 Aug 2015.

SILVA JA, MOREIRA EC, HADDAD JPA, MODENA CM, TUBALDINI MAS. **Temporal and special distribution of rabies in Minas Gerais, 1976 to 1997**. Arq. Bras. Med. Vet. Zootec., v.55, n.3, 2001,p.680 to 684.

SILVA RC, LANGONI H, MENOZZI BD, CAMOSSI LG, GRECA JUNIOR HG, CAMARGO LB, FACCIOLI PY. **Maintenance of rabies virus in non-hematophagous bats (**Artibeus lituratus **and** Myotis **spp.) in Botucatu, SP.** Biological, São Paulo 2006: 68;140-142.

Appendix

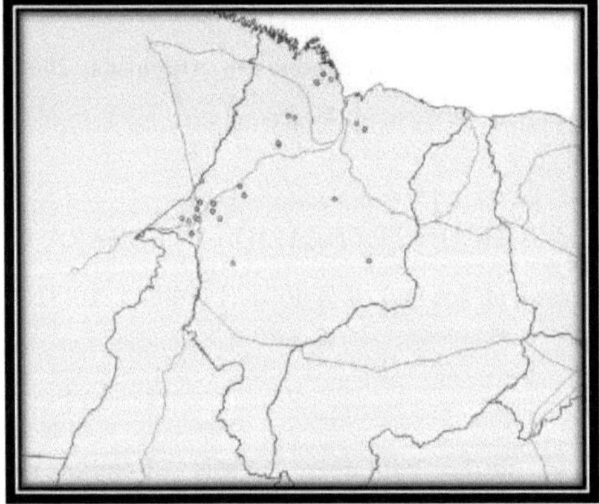

Figura 1. Spatial view of rabies outbreaks (blue pins) and railways (orange lines) at state of Maranhão from 2007 to 2013.

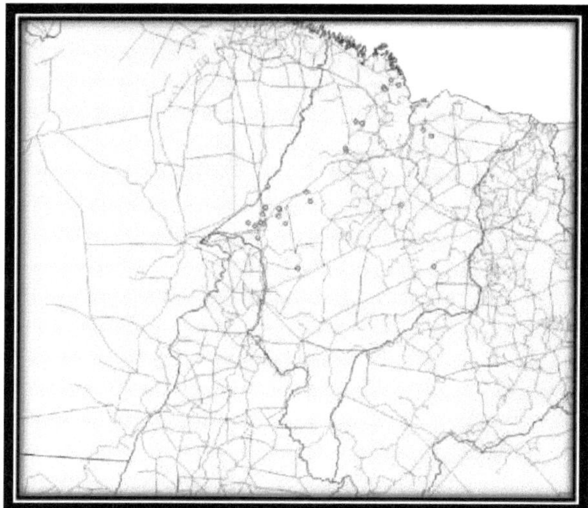

Figura 2. Spatial view of rabies outbreaks (blue pins), railways (orange lines) and roads (green lines) in the state of Maranhão from 2007 to 2013.

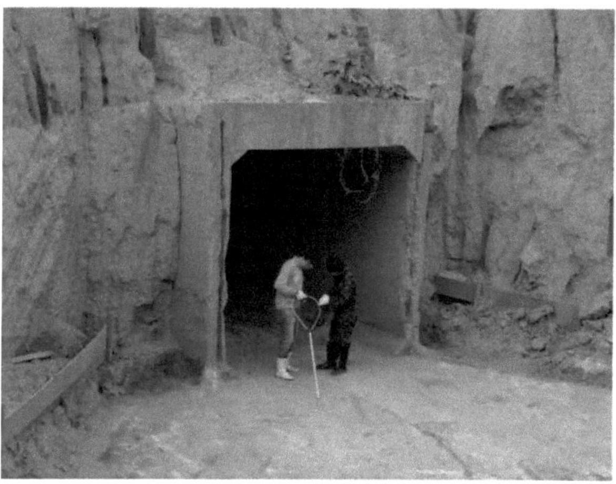

Figura 3. Image of a tunnel on the Carajás Railway **Photo:** Cleide Cunha

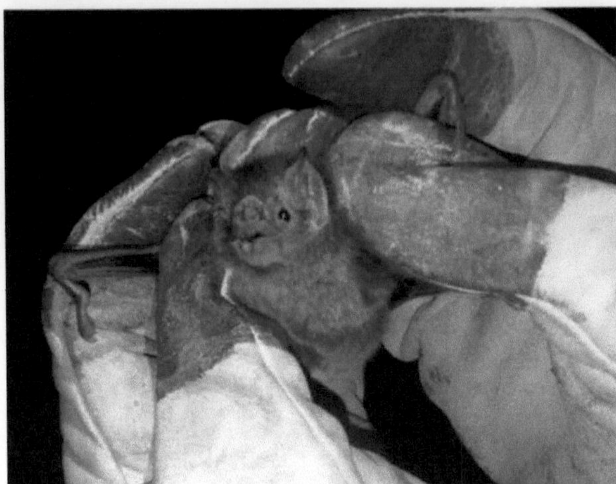

Figura 4. Desmodus rotundus captured in a tunnel on the Carajás Railway

Photo: Damião Renildo

CHAPTER 4

EVALUATION OF THE TEMPORAL AND SPATIAL OCCURRENCE OF RABIES IN HERBIVORES IN THE MICRO-REGION OF CODÓ / MARANHÃO - BRAZIL

Roberto Carlos Negreiros de Arruda [1], José Carlos Pereira de Souza[1], Elaine Fátima de Sena [1], Francisca Neide Costa [2], Hamilton Pereira Santos [2], Helder de Moraes Pereira [2], Sonivalde Santana Monte [3], Humberto de Campos [3] Salim Jorge Waquim [4], Helena Beatriz de Carvalho Ruthner Batista [5]

Summary:

With the aim of evaluating the spatial occurrence of herbivore rabies in the Codó micro-region in Maranhão, we analysed data on notifications in all hematophagous bat control forms and disease investigation forms (MAPA/AGED-MA model) issued between 2004 and 2008. Analysis of the results showed that of the three existing species of haematophagous bats, D. rotundus is the most common vampire in the region. The clinical signs observed in the 16 outbreak properties were: altered behaviour, ataxia, absence of pupillary reflex, head tilted to one side, lateral decubitus, flaccidity of the tail, fever, involuntary movements, pedal movements, mydriasis, nystagmus, opisthotomy, paralysis of the thoracic and pelvic limbs, altered psyche, tenesmus and sialorrhoea. As for the outbreaks of rabies in herbivores in the Codó micro-region, there was a progression of rabies in the order of 95.29 km^2/year. In view of these results, it can be concluded that better veterinary care with effective measures to control outbreaks of rabies, combined with health education actions to raise community awareness, would minimise the progression of outbreaks, since the veterinarian's work at the index outbreak reduces the number of cattle killed per property.

Keywords: Rabies, herbivores, clinical signs and Desmudus rotundus

[1] Federal Agricultural Inspector of the Ministry of Agriculture, Livestock and Food Supply (Maranhão/Brazil)

[2] State University of Maranhão - UEMA

[3] Maranhão State Agricultural Defence Agency - AGED/MA.

[4] Maranhão State Health Secretariat

[5] Federal University of Rio Grande do Sul (UFRGS), RS Brazil

Introduction

Rabies is a zoonosis caused by a virus that infects domestic and wild animals. It is transmitted to other animals and humans through the inoculation of viral particles contained in the saliva of infected animals (bites, scratches, licks or lesions on the skin and mucous membranes). Once the signs of the disease are evident, rabies is fatal to humans and animals (WHO, 2008). Mammals include mainly carnivores and chiropterans (RUPPRECHT et al., 2008). Rabies is present on all continents and is endemic in most African and Asian countries. It is estimated that each year it causes the death of more than 40,000 human beings worldwide (WHO, 2008).

With the aim of standardising control actions, the Ministry of Agriculture set up the Plan to Combat Herbivore Rabies in 1966. This plan has now been restructured through specific legislation and since 2002 has been called the National Herbivore Rabies Control Programme (PNCRH) (BRASIL, 2005). Analysis by the Maranhão Agricultural Health Service (SEDESA/MA) in 2008 showed that between 1987 and 2007, 60,931 outbreaks of rabies in herbivores were recorded in the country, an average of 5,539.18 per year, of which 88.86% were in cattle. However, even with the population of susceptible species increasing, the number of outbreaks has been falling (MAPA, 2008).

Despite the advances in control and prophylaxis systems seen in recent decades, especially with regard to human rabies transmitted by dogs, this zoonosis is still a public health problem in the state of Maranhão. In terms of domestic herbivores, there are 7 million ruminants in the state. Maranhão's livestock industry has a number of health problems, among which rabies stands out, either because of the considerable direct and indirect economic damage caused by the mortality of herbivores (FEITAL & CONFALONIERI, 1998), or because of the potential risk to public health, characterised by the confirmed viral circulation in reported outbreaks. In addition to mortality in cattle, haematophagous bats have contributed to the high number of deaths in humans caused by variant 3 (D. rotundus). In 2005 alone, there were 24 deaths, 17 in the municipality of Turiaçú, 3 in Godofredo Viana, 2 in Cândido Mendes and 2 in Carutapera (ARRUDA et al, 2007).

With a view to tackling the rabies problem in Maranhão, characterised by the episodes that occurred in humans in 2004 and 2005, efforts were intensified between the State University of Maranhão (UEMA), the Maranhão State Agricultural Defence Agency (AGED/MA), Secretary of State for Health (SES/MA) and the Ministry of Agriculture (MAPA/SFA/MA), to strengthen interactive measures, prioritising team training for actions to control herbivore rabies, with a focus on controlling transmitters and immunising susceptible species and paying attention to outbreaks of canine rabies. Although these actions were intensified in 2004 and 2005 due to the occurrence of human cases, they began in the municipality of Imperatriz/MA in 2002, when specific training sessions were organised.

The aim of this study was to carry out a retrospective spatial and temporal analysis of outbreaks of rabies in herbivores in the municipality of Codó Maranhão between 2004 and 2008, focusing on the transmitting species, clinical signs in suspected animals and the spread of the rabies virus in the micro-region studied.

Material and method

Information on animal rabies from 2004 to 2008 was obtained by consulting haematophagous bat control forms and epidemiological investigation and disease notification forms (MAPA model) issued by technicians from the Maranhão State Agricultural Defence Agency during that period. We identified the coordinates of the properties where events were recorded, specifically outbreaks of rabies in herbivores, and which were attended by doctors veterinarians from the official service of the Codó regional unit. TrackMaker and Google Earth® were used to spatially analyse the events, using the coordinates of the properties' headquarters. In addition to the epidemiological investigation into the occurrence of the disease, semi-structured interviews were carried out with the owners or people responsible, in accordance with Minayo, 2004, where, among other things, questions were asked about the clinical signs observed during the care of animals whose samples came back positive, the types of shelters found, vaccinations, and the number of animals killed by species. The spread of rabies outbreaks in herbivores in the Codó micro-region was assessed using the MapSource programme and the Geotastistics for the Environmental Sciences (GS+) ® programme was also used to simulate the absence of assistance and quantify the outbreaks in the study area in the absence of official veterinary assistance.

Results and discussion

Despite the diversification of susceptible species on the farms in the Codó micro-region, 161 pigs, 103 goats, 235 sheep, 43 horses, 161 mules and 1,273 cattle were observed. Only in the last group were deaths recorded, with 35 deaths from rabies reported (2.74%) of the total. This leads to the inference that cattle are the main source of food in terms of quantity and body mass for Desmodus rotundus in the region. Corroborating this inference is the fact that when analysing the data from properties with rabies reports, 45.75% reported the presence of bites from haematophagous bats in cattle, suggesting that rabies transmitted by these bats basically depends on the presence of the virus in the colony. These observations were similar to those reported by GONÇALVES et *al.* (2002) when he stated that "outbreaks of attacks by haematophagous bats on human beings seem to be a common phenomenon in many regions of Latin America, but the occurrence of human rabies transmitted by bats is low".

Looking at the reports of raids caused by D. rotundus and outbreaks of human and animal rabies in 2005 in the north-western region of the state of Maranhão, it was confirmed that these occurrences took place in an area where there were few domestic herbivores and wild animals disappeared due to anthropogenic action. In the micro-region of Codó, this was not observed, since there were no attacks on humans. In relation to the density of the municipality's cattle population, 1.28 cattle/ha, it was observed that bites from haematophagous bats occurred where there was little food on offer for Desmodus rotundus, unlike, for example, what was observed in Imperatriz, where there were 63.68 cattle/ha, and no human attacks were reported, an observation that differs from those reported in Godofredo Viana/MA, where people were found to have been attacked.

Of the 16 bovine CNS samples sent by the veterinarian at the AGED-MA Local Veterinary Care Unit in the municipality of Codó to the rabies diagnostic laboratory at the State University of Maranhão between 2004 and 2008, 10 (62%) were positive for rabies. In addition to the cattle, a haematophagous bat of the species D. rotundus and an unidentified non-hematophagous bat also reacted. When comparing these results with the occurrences of rabies in herbivores recorded throughout Maranhão between 2004 and 2007, when 19 outbreaks were confirmed in 2004, 25 in 2005, 31 in 2006 and 12 in 2007, it was observed that cattle were the most affected, with 89%, 84%, 64% and 92% respectively. BARBOSA E COSTA (1997), cited outbreaks of rabies with high mortality rates in foxes of the Cerdocyon thous species, reporting attacks on nine people in the municipality of Timon and one in Caxias. It should be emphasised that to this day fox rabies is very common in this region between Maranhão and Piauí, known as the cocais region, which is part of the Codó micro-region (figure 1). As well as haematophagous bats, foxes are blamed for attacking animals in this area, including domestic herbivores, and this species is also considered to spread the disease. This corroborates the reports by GOMES in 2004, when he cited that the northeastern fox is a wild reservoir of the rabies virus in the semi-arid region of Paraíba, in the municipality of Patos, and is pathogenic for goats, sheep, horses, donkeys and mice, showing biological behaviour compatible with the classic sample of the rabies virus. SPINDOLA et al (2006) reported that in 2005, in the state of Piauí, several animals of the Cerdocion thous species were found to be infected with the rabies virus.

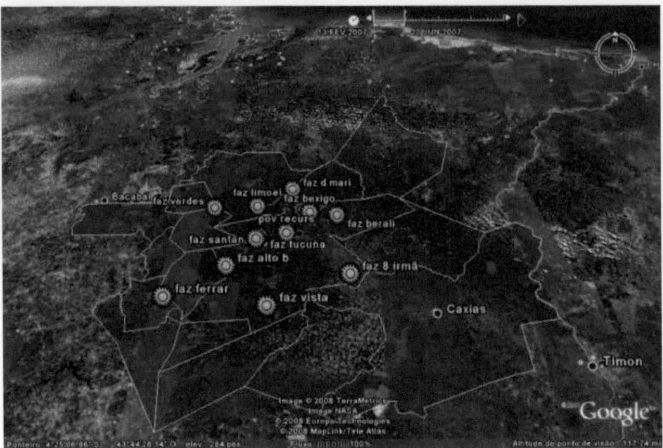

Figura 1 - Map: view of rabies outbreaks in herbivores in the babassu region (Codó micro-region) between 2004 and 2008. Source: GoogleEarth.

The three species of haematophagous bats Diphylla ecaudata, Diaemus youngi, and D. rotundus have already been found in the state of Maranhão, but Desmodus rotundus is the most common species in the babassu region.

In 2007, technicians from the Defence Agency captured 365 haematophagous bats throughout the state, of which 931 were captured and treated, i.e. an average of close to 3 (three) specimens per capture. These captures are normally made in corrals, however, in the Codó micro-region, from observations on the haematophagous bat control forms, this number rose to 5 (five) bats. In the micro-region studied, houses, abandoned wells, hollow sticks, caves, caves and culverts on roads and railways were identified as artificial shelters. These were rarely captured. In Codó, 6 (six) Desmodus were caught in an abandoned well attacking pigs 200 metres from the farmers' homes.

Among the outbreaks of rabies in herbivores in the babassu area of the Codó Microregion, between February 2005 and July 2008, it was observed that cattle were the species affected. In this outbreak area, there was a diagram of 6,279.00 km^2 between the outbreaks, so considering the perimeter of the polygon between the equidistant points in a straight line, a polygon of 349.4 km^2 was formed in 44 months, i.e. an evolution of 95.29 km(2) per year (Figure 2).

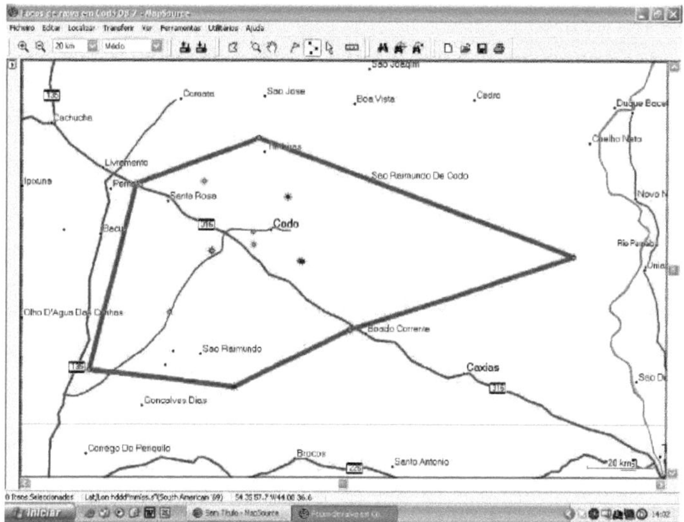

Figura 2 - Map: diagram of rabies outbreaks in herbivores in the Cocais Region (Codó Microregion) between 2004 and 2008, presented in the MapSource programme.

In the area studied, there was also a high level of cattle mortality when the outbreaks were assessed, so using the Geostatistics for the Environmental Sciences (GS+) programme, the risk of spread was estimated if there was no official veterinary assistance for the outbreaks in the area. The average number of cattle killed per property was 2.29 animals, with a maximum of 13 (thirteen) cattle and a minimum of 1 (one), out of a total of 35 animals. When the cause of the higher number of animals on one property and the low mortality on others was assessed, it was inferred how important the veterinary doctor's guidance is in controlling the index outbreak or outbreak, when compared to a previous outbreak, given that four months had passed between the deaths and the first veterinary visit (Figure 3).

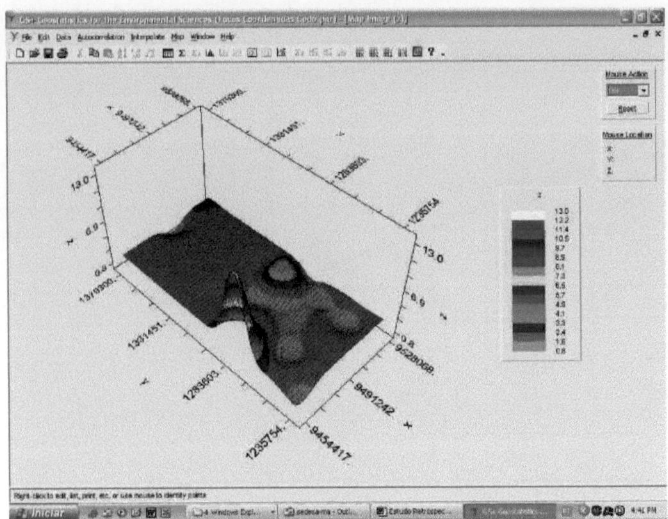

Figura 3 - Graph: Risk calculated by the Geostatistics for the Environmental Sciences (GS+) programme in the area studied if there is no official veterinary assistance for outbreaks.

Analysing the information on clinical signs in sick herbivores in the micro-region, it was observed that death was always preceded by behavioural and balance disorders. The clinical signs observed were: ataxia with staggering gait, absence of pupillary reflex, head tilted to one side, lateral decubitus, flaccidity of the tail, involuntary movements, pedal movements, mydriasis, opisthotomy, paralysis of the pelvic limbs, paralysis of the thoracic limbs, altered psyche reflected when the animal is not alert to its surroundings, tenesmus or continuous effort to urinate or defecate and sialorrhoea. These clinical manifestations were similar to those reported by HIPOLITO et al. (1965), CORREA (1970), ACHA & SZIFRES (1986), BLOOD & HENDERSON (1978), PITZSCHKE (1988). The signs observed in the visits varied according to the stage of the disease at the time of the vet's visit to the property, as the animals were not always observed every day and some reflexes were not tested in the clinical assessment. Despite being included in the questionnaire, no questions were answered about manifestations of: aggression, absence of anal reflex, bruxism, blindness, sternal decubitus, tongue flaccidity, miosis, hoarse mooing, priapism, pruritus and trismus or paralysis of the jaw. Similar to these observations, BORGES et al (2006) also reported that some signs found in the literature were not observed in their findings, such as: vocal alterations, frequent screaming, aggression, local itching, mutilations, blindness and head pressure on objects.

ARRUDA et al (2007) observed that even though there were no cases of rabies on farms in Caxias/MA, a city close to the region studied, 82% of the farmers interviewed vaccinated their animals, but did not booster vaccinate them after 30 days, according to technical instructions. They also observed that 62% of those interviewed did not use any measures against attacks by haematophagous bats, while 25% of those interviewed used unconventional control methods such as using chilli peppers on the wounds made by haematophagous bats.

With regard to the outbreaks attended in the micro-region, it was noted that even though they were instructed to do so, vaccination boosters were almost never given 21 to 30 days after the first vaccination, leaving the animals immunologically unprotected. It is also important to emphasise the importance of sucking up animals under 3 months old, which are not protected by colostrum due to the lack of mother vaccination. It is therefore suggested that livestock farmers be better informed about the need for booster vaccinations in foci and perifocal areas, as this practice was observed to be inconsistent, and that they should be warned about the use of vampiricide on animals that have been attacked in regions where there have been reports of attacks by haematophagous bats. On the other hand, he drew attention to the need for better veterinary attention to the index focus, which would certainly reduce the number of cattle killed. Special attention should also be paid to the northeastern fox as an important reservoir of wild rabies in northeastern Brazil, emphasising the identification of the viral variant circulating in this species.

References

ACHA, P.N.; SZYFRES,B. **Zoonoses and transmissible diseases common to humans and animals.** 2. ed. Washington: PAHO/WHO, 1986.

AMORIM, A. M.; SOUZA J. C. S.; PICCININI, R. S. **Clinical and laboratory diagnosis of rabies in horses: A warning for clinicians.** The XV

International Conference Rabies in the Americas XV RITA. Santo Domingo, Dominican

Republic. Abstracts Book, p 62, 2004.

ARRUDA, R. C. N. de. **Educational diagnosis on rabies in the municipality of Caxias, Maranhão.** Citation of reports. Agricultural Health Service - SEDESA/SFA/MA. São Luís. 2006. 18p.

ARRUDA, R. C. N. de; GOULART; C. da S; MARQUES, G. H. F; SOUZA, J. C. P. de; SILVEIRA, P. P.; SANTOS, H. P.; MONTE, S. S.; WAQUIM, S. J.; MARTINS, J. O. de S.; FILHO, H. C. M.; Rabies diagnosis in domestic herbivorous in Caxias, Maranhão, Brazil. **Annal - International Conference Rabies in Americas. Permanent Post Session.** Guanajuato. Mexico. 29th September - 5th October 2007.

ARRUDA, R. C. N. de; GOULART; C. da S; MARQUES, G. H. F; SOUZA, J. C. P. de; SILVEIRA, P. P.; SANTOS, H. P.; MONTE, S. S.; WAQUIM, S. J.; MARTINS, J. O. de S.; FILHO, H. C. M.; Misuse of Carbamate (aldicarb) in skin lesions caused by vampire bats in Godofredo Viana, Maranhão, Brazil. **Annal - International Conference Rabies in Americas. Permanent Post Session.** Guanajuato. Mexico. 29th September - 5th October 2007.

BARBOSA, A. dos S.; COSTA, R. de O. **Notification of attacks by foxes** Pseudalopex vetulus (D. vetulus) **on people and animals in Timon and Caxias, Maranhão**. Report. Timon Zoonosis Control Centre - CCZ. 1997. 3p.

BORGES, J. R.; MOSCARDINI, A. R. C.; COST, L. M. C. C.; BREDT, A.; NETO TEIXEIRA A. R.; CUNHA, P. H. J. Clinical Aspect of rabies in bovine in the Centre-West of Brazil. **Annal - International Conference Rabies in Americas.** Brasília. Brazil. 15th-20th october 2006. 220p.

BLOOD, D.C.; HENDERSON, J.A. **Veterinary Medicine.** 4. ed. Rio de Janeiro: Guanabara Koogan, 1978.

BRAZIL. Ministry of Agriculture, Livestock and Supply. **Control of herbivore rabies.** Brasília: MAPA/SDA/DSA. 2005. 104p.

CORRÊA, O. **Infectious diseases of domestic animals.** Rio de Janeiro: Freitas Bastos, v.3, 1970.

FEITAL, A. S. S.; CONFALONIERI, U. E. C. **Epidemiological study of bovine rabies in the State of Rio de Janeiro, Brazil (1980-1992).** Revista Brasileira de Ciência Veterinária, v5, n.1, 21-27, jan./abr.1998.

GOMES, A. A. de B.; **Epidemiology of rabies: characterisation of viruses isolated from domestic and wild animals in the semi-arid region of Patos, Paraiba.** PhD thesis. USP. São Paulo. 2004. 107p.

GONÇALVES, M. A. S.; SÁ-NETO, R. J.; BRAZIL, T. K. **Outbreak of aggressions and transmission of rabies in human beings by vampire bats in**

northeastern Brazil. Journal of the Brazilian Society of Tropical Medicine. 35(5): 461-464, Sep-Oct, 2002.

HIPÓLITO, O.; FREITAS, M.G. FIGUEIREDO, J.B. **Doenças Infecto- Contagiosas dos Animais Domésticos.** 4. ed. Local: Melhoramentos, 1965.

MINAYO, M.C.S. **O desafio do conhecimento: pesquisa qualitativa em saúde**. São Paulo - Rio de Janeiro: ABRASCO-HUCITEC, 2004. 269p.

MINISTRY OF AGRICULTURE, LIVESTOCK AND SUPPLY. Spreadsheets from the Coordination of the National Programme for the Control of Herbivore Rabies and other Encephalopathies - PNCRH. Brasília: MAPA/SDA/DSA. 2008.

WORLD HEALTH ORGANISATION, 2008. Rabia Justification of surveillance. [online] Available on the Internet via http://www.paho.org/spanish/sha/be_v21n3-casos.htm#rabia. Accessed on 19 July, 2008.

PITZSCHKE, H. Rabies. IN: BEER, J. **Infectious Diseases in Domestic Animals.** Place: publisher.V.1, 1988.

RUPPRECHT C. H; HANLON C. A; HEMACHUDHA T.; **Rabies re-examined.** Available on the Internet via WWW. URL: http://www.ncbi.nlm.nih.gov/pubmed/12144896. Accessed 19 June, 2008.

SPINDOLA, R. O.; SILVA, J. P. da; CARVALHO, R. C. de; CARVALHO, V. M. A.; ACHKAR, S. M. CASTILHO, J. G.; CERETTA, R. S.; KOTAIT, I. Investigation of rabies virus in the salivary glands of wild dogs (Cerdocion thurs),

naturally infected in the state of Piauí. **Annal - International Conference Rabies in Americas.** Brasilia. Brazil. 15th-20th october 2006. 220p.

[WHO] WORLD HEALTH ORGANISATION; Rabies; [online] Available from Internet via WWW. URL: http://www.who.int/mediacentre/factsheets/fs099/en/. Accessed on 19 June, 2008.

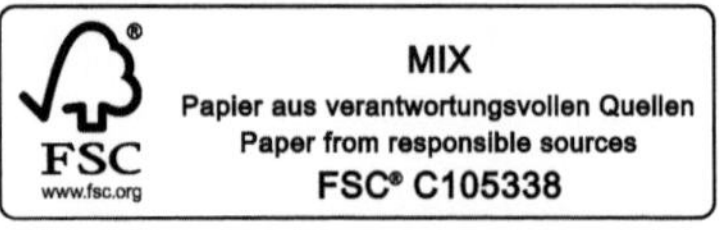

Printed by Books on Demand GmbH, Norderstedt / Germany